INTRODUCTION TO CELL BIOLOGY AND EPIGENETICS

INTRODUCTION FO CELL BIOLOGY AND EPIGENETICS

Introduction to Cell Biology and Epigenetics

Kelly Gregg MD

INTRODUCTION FO CELL BIOLOGY AND EPIGENETICS

Copyright 2021by Kelly Gregg

All Rights Reserved

ISBN 979-875-979-0648

Kelly.ewriter@gmail.com

Kellygregg.com

TABLE OF CONTENTS

Introduction	7
Cell Membrane	13
Cell biology	27
Cell Nucleus	37
DNA	47
RNA	61
Chromosomes	79
Methylation	89
Virus	107
Epigenetics	115
Diet and Health	129

INTRODUCTION FO CELL BIOLOGY AND EPIGENETICS

INTRODUCTION

Many of you have studied my book *Diet and Health,* and some of you may have completed all the study and graduated with a college degree. Now we are going to graduate school. I will be writing about *Epigenetics in Diet and Health.*

Unlike the study of diet and your health, in which most of us have practical knowledge just based upon life experience, this subject may not be as familiar to you. Like my previous book in which I had to make sure everyone knew about metabolism and nutrition, which required my teaching you the basics; I am going to have to teach you some basics of cell biology and genetics for you to understand the subject. Most of you learned some of this in high school and, if you are like the average person, you promptly forgot as it had little use in your life. I am going to remind you of what you learned and add a little to it. If you did not graduate from high school, it does not make any difference as I am going to teach you anyway.

Like my previous book I will write this in several small books and combine them all at the end. This is the way the economics of Kindle Direct Publishing works. Along the way I will provide audiobooks for those who are too lazy to read.

Currently *Epigenetics in Diet and Health* is going to be composed of three books. This one, *Introduction to Cell Biology and Epigenetics*, the next, E*pigenetics and Pregnancy: Fat Newborns and Kids* which is already published, and the next one not yet published being *Epigenetics and the Gut Biome.* Since this is a graduate course, it will be harder than the previous book; but that is mainly because I must teach you the lingo. Your common sense is adequate once you understand the language.

Do not hold me to this exact outline. It's the same as when you write fiction books. Once you start writing, the plot may take you anywhere.

I have concluded that genetics plays a minor role in Diet and Health and is not a major factor in epigenetics. That is not to say your genetics may have a major role in your overall health, but it is not a factor over which you have any control. Your diet for most of your life is controlled by you. That is something you can change.

Upon finishing this current book, it ended up be slightly more technical than I thought it would be. I have edited it but do not believe I can decrease the technical parts without depriving you of necessary information. I have a high opinion of your common sense and think you can understand it.

INTRODUCTION FO CELL BIOLOGY AND EPIGENETICS

With the advent of Covid over the last few years, I have added a chapter on Viruses. This will give you some basic information as to how viruses work. I did use the Covid virus as an example, but most of the information will apply to most viruses.

I have written a much more detailed book entitled Covid and Vaccines for the Common Man in which I talk much more about the virus, the vaccine, the disease, and to some extent the politics. At this point we cannot separate government from science from media. A decade ago I trusted the CDC and the FDA. Now I do not. Now Amazon will not allow me to advertise my book on covid, although most is just basic science, or vaccines, although most is just a discussion of the immune system.

I hope the few sentences I write on the covid virus do not taint this entire book and get it banned from advertising on Amazon.

I am left with trying to educate you enough that you can understand what the government and media is saying and use your common sense to make intelligent decisions for you and your family.

INTRODUCTION FO CELL BIOLOGY AND EPIGENETICS

Chapter One
Cell Membrane

We are going to start with cell biology. Most of you have some knowledge of what a cell is. You either learned it in school or picked it up somewhere in your life experiences. Most of the things you learn in life are not in school. If you can read, you can learn almost anything, especially now that Google exists.

    I am going to teach you the basics of what is a cell and what is inside. . You probably already knew some about human chromosomes, and I will eventually refresh your memory about them.

    If I ask someone to visualize or draw a cell, they will usually think of something like a marble. Perhaps because often, we see pictures of white blood cells on TV, or perhaps a picture of a human egg cell. Most of our cells do not really look like marbles.

Think of your brain cells or neurons. Nothing like a marble. Heart, muscle liver, kidney, and all the other organs are not marble like. The cells lining the gut may be more rectangular than round. The round cells are often found in the liquid in your body like the blood. The most common cell in the blood is the red blood cell which is more disc-like. The white cells are usually round, but they represent a small portion of the cells in the blood.

I am going to follow the crowd and represent the cell as a marble because it is easy to draw, and easier to represent the contents by imagining a circle. Remember this is not real life. I will sometimes speak about the size of a cell and may mention a diameter. This does not mean the cell is round and I really mean the average size, not the diameter. In all cells the size changes a little all the time, depending on the environment.

Things enter into the cells, and this is part of the cause of epigenetics. Your cells are usually in a somewhat liquid environment, even those cells not in the blood. Environment includes things like temperature or pH of the surrounding fluid. It also includes the varying concentration of all the different ions that may be present. It also involves all the various chemicals and compounds we are exposed to daily. Things that touch our skin, things we eat, things in the air we breathe, even things produced by other organisms that may be inside us or in our gut. We are continuously exposed to factors that may cause epigenetic changes. It appears these changes can occur with exposure to very small amounts of these substances. I'm talking about way less than parts per trillion. Levels are so small we are unable to measure them.

INTRODUCTION FO CELL BIOLOGY AND EPIGENETICS

I guess it is time to define what epigenetics is. The most common definition is:

Heritable changes in gene expression that do not involve changes in the underlying DNA sequence. Almost all of these changes are not inherited in the next generation but are passed on to the next cell when it undergoes mitosis.

Most of us know a little something about genes. We know we have DNA in us which makes up chromosomes. We know there are two sets of chromosomes in the cell, and that with reproduction, one set of chromosomes from the male combines with one set from the female and forms a new combined set of chromosomes. This is sexual reproduction and true for almost all animals. Bacteria reproduce by simply duplicating their chromosomes and do not combine two different sets of chromosomes.

We also know that sometimes when cells duplicate themselves the process goes awry. The resultant cell has an error in the DNA such that the subsequent cell divisions also have this error. This we call a mutation. If this occurs in sperm or egg cells, this error can be passed on to the next generation.

Epigenetics concerns itself with the expression of the DNA withing the cell. We innately know that all our cells which have a nucleus contain a copy of all our chromosomes (not sperm or egg, they only have half). So theoretically every cell should be able to produce any other cell, including duplicating every part of the cell from which it came from.

Obviously, this does not happen randomly as we have many different types of cells in the body, despite their all having the same DNA. It's just that this DNA is expressed differently.

INTRODUCTION FO CELL BIOLOGY AND EPIGENETICS

Epigenetics does concern itself with development, but I am going to mainly talk about what happens after development. The environment can change the expression of some of the genes, without changing the DNA itself. It turns out this is quite important.

Identical twins start out with the same DNA, and when they get old, they still have the same DNA, but they end up not the same. The DNA has been expressed differently, and the environment is responsible for this different expression. This occurs in all of us and the environment in which the cells are exposed is primarily responsible. The change in the expression of our genes goes on throughout our life. It is quite dynamic and sometimes the change is rapid.

The goal of this book is to explore and explain how our diet affects these changes, and how this affects our health. I must teach you a bunch of other stuff in order for you to understand what I am talking about.

This same process occurs in bacteria, and our gut biome changes as we are exposed to a particular diet. Not only our diet, but other things that happen to get into what we eat, like insecticides or environmental pollutants. It may change our body cells somewhat, but it may change our gut bacteria in a different way.

One of my favorite examples concerns honeybees. The queen bee is much larger than the normal working bee. In the hive, most all the bees are female workers. There is only one queen. The queen has a well-developed reproductive system and lays 2000 eggs a day. These are all fertilized eggs. All the female worker bees have almost the same DNA as the queen bee, yet rarely can they lay eggs, and these are not fertilized. An unfertilized egg becomes a male bee (drone) with only half the chromosomes of a female bee.

INTRODUCTION FO CELL BIOLOGY AND EPIGENETICS

    A queen bee starts out as a normal worker egg that the nurse bees feed a large amount of royal jelly secreted by head glands. This is a concentrated mixture of proteins, amino acids, unusual lipids vitamins, and other unknown compounds. All the bee eggs get a little of this, but the larvae destined to be a queen get a huge amount. The queen continues to be fed with royal jelly, with constant grooming, and protection by the worker bees. Her life span will be at least 20 times longer than a worker.

    All of these changes are epigenetic, produced by her diet. Her chromosomes are the same as all the other worker bee eggs that were laid by the new queens mother. This is an example of a diet producing changes in the expression of the DNA, but not changing the DNA.

    Of course, we don't have the equivalent of royal jelly, and even if that were all you ate, you would not live twenty times longer. Although eating a diet very high in these types of elements probably would cause some epigenetic changes.

I will mention epigenetics almost every chapter. After all, this is the title of the series.

Back to the cell. I will start with the cell membrane which separates the inside of the cell from the outside. Animal cells to not have a cell wall. Plants do. Most bacteria do. The cell wall is not the cell membrane, although bacteria have both. We call bacteria cell membranes the plasma membrane.

Like everything in your body, this is quite complicated. Those of you who have read *Diet and Health* know that I believe in creation, as the more you understand the human body, or any living organism, you realize how unbelievably complicated is the interaction among all its elements. So much so that it appears impossible that this could have developed spontaneously. The cell membrane is no exception.

The membrane is mainly composed of two lipid layers, actually phospholipids, which means that one end of the molecule repels water (hydrophobic) whereas the other end of the molecule, which is on the inside of these two layers, likes water (hydrophilic). This makes the inside of the membrane fluid. There are other components such as cholesterol (which stiffens the membrane), carbohydrates, and various other proteins.

The membrane separates the cell from the environment but must allow transport of all kinds of things to the inside to maintain homeostasis. Energy is required which means glucose, fatty acids, and ketone bodies must have access to the inside of the cell. Various chemical ions and water must also penetrate. Some of these, like water, may be driven by osmotic pressure. The membrane has ion gates which can control how many ions may pass. The membrane can also engulf various elements in a vesicle composed of a different type of membrane, and transport this to the cytoplasm. It can do the opposite and allow vesicles to be transported out of the cell, like hormones, or say insulin. Vacuoles are combined vesicles and are usually filled with water. These membranes are also formed of phospholipids.

On the outside of the cell membrane are numerous receptors. These are ligands, which means they are attached to the membrane on one end, and usually attached to a larger protein on the other end. They are usually quite specific and there are hundreds of different kinds of receptors around the cell, and thousands of each receptor (10,00-20,000) Think of a beach ball covered with fuzz. Once attached, complicated reactions then occur which can cause changes inside the cell and selectively change the permeability of the membrane. It may cause the cell membrane to form a vesicle which will engulf the ligand and transport it to the cytoplasm. Things going in and out of the cell is happening continuously and it is a complicated process to maintain homeostasis in the cell. Many of these reactions happen in microseconds.

I mention all this because this is the way epigenetics occurs. The environment outside the cell affects the inside of the cell, not only in the cytoplasm, but also in the nucleoplasm which is inside the nuclear membrane.

You may remember talking about the gut membrane in a previous book which must keep harmful things out of your body yet let many things in the food you eat into the body. Nowadays everyone is familiar with the spike proteins on the corona virus which must interact with a receptor on the cell membrane to enter the cell.

As you can see, the membrane is a very active environment which is continuously transporting things in and out. It is made by DNA and organelles in the cell. The membrane transports elements that can lead to different expressions of your DNA or can lead to effects on the cell membrane itself to affect what enters. There is a continual change in the DNA expression, but the DNA itself is unchanged.

I could go on, but the more we learn, the more complicated it gets. The same is true about every process in the body, which by the way is composed of about 30 trillion cells. All with the same DNA, yet all may have a slightly different internal environment. Somehow, they all work together to keep you alive. Oh yeah, you have another 30 trillion bacteria in your gut.

INTRODUCTION FO CELL BIOLOGY AND EPIGENETICS

Chapter Two
Cell Biology

We are going over the biology of the cell to get down some basic lingo. I will refer to these organelles throughout the book, so you need to know what I am talking about.

I have divided the cell into thirds. We just covered the cell membrane. Now I am going to talk about the space between the cell membrane and the nuclear membrane. Then we will go over the nucleus.

Outside the cell is the environmental stuff that causes epigenetic changes. Inside the cell membrane is the cytoplasm where much of the epigenetic changes occur, as well as the production of the proteins that are being changed. This is where much of the RNA lives. Inside the nucleus is where the DNA resides. Epigenetic changes do not change the DNA but does change the expression of the DNA. The DNA makes the RNA which travels into the cytoplasm. I will talk a lot more about DNA and RNA later, really most of the book.

The cytoplasm is mostly water, about 80%. It is in this milieu where biochemical reactions take place. There are several structures within, and we will go over them.

First is the cytoskeleton. I do not recall anyone ever teaching me about this, from high school through college. It is not particularly exciting but quite necessary. Don't worry if you have never heard of it because 98% of the people haven't either.

The cytoskeleton is a complex network of protein filaments that span the cytoplasm, from the cell membrane to the nucleus, from one cell membrane to another and between the organelles. It also associates with extracellular connective tissue to stabilize cells throughout the body. These filaments are always changing and capable of rapidly forming and disassembling.

We usually divide these into three types: microfilaments, intermediate filaments, and microtubules. Microfilaments are made of actin, one of the most abundant proteins in your body, and capable of interacting will all kinds of other proteins. These are not just strings but are metabolically active and are involved in muscle contraction, moving things around in the cell, and changing the shape of the cell membrane.

Intermediate filaments are slightly larger and composed of several other types of proteins. They are involved in the anchoring of organelles in the cell. You do not want everybody to pile up on one side of the cell.

Microtubules are the largest and, as you would guess, are involved in moving things around. They bind to many components and enable the organelles to move around. If you have cells with cilia, these are composed of microtubules.

Vacuoles are membranes which enclose things, all kinds of things, and are present throughout the cytoplasm. These are types of vesicle. Both are membrane enclosed organelles, although vacuoles usually contain more liquid. Vesicles have a double membrane and contain all kinds of things like solids, various molecules, maybe bacteria, or all kinds of things. The membrane of a vacuole does not combine with other membranes, unlike the vesicle. A vesicle can combine with a vacuole. The cell membrane can invaginate and surround things in a vesicle to transport it into the cytoplasm, or it can do the reverse. There are lots of them in the cytoplasm. If you recall *Diet and Health*, you have lysosomes, which are full of enzymes and chemicals, are classified as a type of vacuole which can fuse with a vesicle.

    The endoplasmic reticulum is a bunch of flat tubes folded upon itself and associated with the nuclear membrane. It exists in two forms: the rough endoplasmic reticulum and the smooth. They exist close to each other and by the nucleus, but spreads throughout the cytoplasm. We call one rough because it is studded with ribosomes on the outside of this flattened tube. I will talk about ribosomes in a minute, but they construct protein out of amino acids for the body. Once a protein is constructed, it is passed into the lumen of the rough endoplasmic reticulum to be modified by folding or the addition of carbohydrates. This is then passed to the Golgi apparatus. The smooth reticulum makes lipid and as such does not have ribosomes stuck to the outside.

Ribosomes are free in the cytoplasm. When mRNA binds to a ribosome, it then attaches to the endoplasmic reticulum to make a specific protein, then it leaves to be replaced by another.

I am going to have a chapter about RNA and DNA. There are lots of different kinds of RNA and I will end up listing them for you. It ends up that RNA is the major player in epigenetics. DNA gives you the general plans, RNA is involved in all the particulars. Practically all your cells have the same DNA, the RNA directs which cells are liver cells or skin cells. The first 16 to 32 cells you have look alike. We can take one out and there is no problem. RNA is responsible for the development of these cells and can them to turn into anything including specific cell types.

Let us move on. I think this may be boring some of you, but only a little bit more. We are learning the lingo and I will refer to some of these structures later. If I wanted to teach you algebra, we would have to go over division. Those of you who already know this, skip to the next chapter. The rest of you hang in there.

The Golgi apparatus is next to the reticulum and receives the manufactured products from the endoplasmic reticulum. It then may modify them somewhat, but primarily forms them into vesicles which are then transported to other parts of the cytoplasm, or perhaps excreted through the cell membrane.

Finally, we have the mitochondria. These are double membrane structures in the cell, usually between 10-200. Many of us remember them to be the energy producing organelles of the cell. Most of us do not remember what that means.

You need energy to live, that is you need energy for your cells to function. All our energy comes from what we eat. A plant takes in energy from the sun in the form of photons. It then takes CO2, and water and makes a sugar molecule. We eat the sugar molecule and get out energy.

It takes energy to make sugar, and it releases energy when we break it down. The same with fats and protein. The production of energy is much more efficient if oxygen is present. When the oxygen is limited in the cells, energy can still be produced without mitochondria through the partial breakdown of glucose. We get about 13 times as much energy if we break down product with mitochondria.

What happens to energy. We have a carrier of energy in the adenosine triphosphate molecule. The mitochondria break down food and releases energy. It than uses this energy to convert ADP (adenosine diphosphate) into ATP. Then we can take this ATP to wherever we want and use the breakdown of ATP into ADP to use the energy there.

The mitochondria do all kinds of other things. The outer membrane contains enzymes that modify fats and protein. The mitochondria can change the way it is producing energy to generate heat if needed. It has several functions but for my purposes, I am going to concentrate on its chromosomes.

Although we consider the nucleus to be the home of DNA, the mitochondria have its own. This is one circular chromosome which codes for about 37 genes, nothing compared to our regular DNA chromosomes which code for 30,000.

Like many organelles in the cell, they reproduce independently from cell division. If you need more energy, the mitochondria divide through fission, and the chromosomes are duplicated. When the whole cell divides (mitosis), the nuclear chromosomes are duplicated. I will talk about mitochondrial DNA later, but this is a special organelle.

INTRODUCTION FO CELL BIOLOGY AND EPIGENETICS

Enough of cell biology, although the next chapter will be on the nucleus, home of the DNA. This is a book about epigenetics in *Diet and Health*. As such our focus is going to be on DNA and RNA, which live in the nucleus. The RNA is also scattered all around the cytoplasm. Cell biology is like gross anatomy; it is the first course in medicine as you must learn what a liver is before you can learn about metabolism.

I will revisit some of the comments I have made when it makes more sense to the topic. Cells are made of organelles composed of millions of molecules. A strand of DNA is one molecule, although a giant one.

Chapter Three
Cell Nucleus

I divided the cell into three components: the environment, which is anything outside the cell, the cytoplasm which is divided from the environment by the cell membrane, and the nucleus which is divided from the rest of the cell by the nuclear membrane. The nuclear membrane is not the same as the cell membrane. It does allow various ions or small molecules to enter, but any large molecules must be transported in through nuclear pores in the membrane. It is also a double membrane but unlike the cell membrane. The outside nuclear membrane communicates directly with the Golgi body and is involved in the production of RNA and proteins.

INTRODUCTION FO CELL BIOLOGY AND EPIGENETICS

The DNA is confined to the nucleus. (I know there is a little in the mitochondria), but there is no DNA in the cytoplasm (not counting DNA viruses). You can find DNA in the bloodstream which originates from cells which have undergone apoptosis or disintegrated for some reason. DNA does not last long in the blood and is metabolized by various enzymes.

The DNA membranes, inner and outer, are unrelated to each other unlike the cell membrane. There are various cell products between the two membranes, and it is the inner membrane that is the barrier between the inside of the nucleus and the cytoplasm. Several thousand pores allow large proteins or nucleic acids (RNA) to be transported from the nucleus to the cytoplasm.

Like the cytoskeleton, the nucleus has its own filaments providing structural support and transportation called the nuclear lamina. These filaments bind to the cytoskeleton as well as to the chromosomes. As we will see in a future chapter, the coiled chromosomes are always in motion and freeing up parts to be coded or coiling to be stored. The filaments are not just strings but are metabolically active and constantly reforming as well as transporting structures in the nucleus. You have 46 chromosomes that are usually partially uncoiled and scattered throughout the nucleus constantly undergoing processes that require some stability or movement. The nuclear lamina provides this service.

    We are used to seeing pictures of chromosomes. These appear to be distinctive linear elements. They only look like that in the part of the cell cycle before division of the cell. Most of the time they are linear molecules intertwined or scattered in the nucleus. Chromosomes are the distinct structures we see. Chromatin is coiled and uncoiled DNA, which is complexed with various proteins, mainly histones, which allow the DNA molecules to form tightly coiled strings visible as chromosomes. Almost everything I will be talking about will be occurring in the chromatin. The DNA of a chromosome is one giant molecule. The DNA wraps around a group of eight histone molecules about 1 1/2 times. You can imagine a long string wrapped around a yoyo, separated by a space, and wrapped around another yoyo, and repeated many times. These yoyo strings thing coil around themselves and form a chromatin fiber The fibers then coil together and eventually form the chromosome. It is like making a rope from lots of string.

    Genes are segments of DNA. To get to the gene, you must unwrap a bunch of coils to get to the one segment you want. Then you divide that one segment apart so you can make RNA. Then you take the RNA to a ribosome to make a protein or whatever that segment of DNA coded for. You can see that you eventually must unwrap that segment from the histones to get access to it.

Now is a good time to remind you of the purpose of the whole book. Epigenetics is the expression of a gene. This expression is affected by different molecules, mainly methyl groups, binding to parts of the DNA. This binding is not permanent, although some may be passed on, and the basic DNA remains the same. It is not a mutation which is a change in the nucleic acid base sequence, but it is dynamic and changes depending on your environment. There are several other mechanisms by which this expression can be modified, including changes that occur in the histones which must unravel to let the DNA code a protein, fat, or steroid. There are further modifications up and down the line, including controls of the manifestation of the proteins which occur outside the nucleus at the site of their action.

INTRODUCTION FO CELL BIOLOGY AND EPIGENETICS

    There are lots of things in the environment which affect this. I am going to concern myself with what you eat, and how this affects your health. Those of you who are familiar with my book *Diet and Health* know I talked about inducing certain enzymes and changing a metabolic set point. Now I am going to go into more detail about what is happening. You do not need to know this to know how to eat a proper diet, but an understanding will give you insight, and perhaps motivation, on how to eat. We still are a long way to go on that subject. Remember this is a graduate course, it is a lot harder than your bachelor's degree.

    Let's finish the nucleus. Eukaryotes are cells which have a nucleus, prokaryotes are cells like bacteria which do not have a nucleus. The DNA in bacteria is in a circular form and is in the cytoplasm. I am mainly interested in human cells but will eventually get to the gut biome. RNA is found throughout the cell, DNA in the nucleus although a few small pieces can be in the cytoplasm. Red blood cells do not have a nucleus and are unable to replace any organelles. They only live about 3 months.

    The interior of the nucleus does not contain any membrane structures like the cytoplasm. Chromosomes are evident during replication of the cell, otherwise they are distributed in the nucleus. The largest discrete body in the nucleus is the nucleolus. This is a densely stained area which does not have a membrane. In forms around certain areas of chromosomes and is composed of DNA regions, RNA, and proteins. Ribosomes are manufactured in these areas and the nucleolus vary in size as the demand for ribosomes changes. Remember ribosomes bind mRNA and manufacture proteins. The rough endoplasmic reticulum is covered with ribosomes.

There are other dense bodies observed in the nucleolus. There are one to ten compact structures called Cajal bodies that resemble a ball of twine. They contain RNA and proteins and may serve to modify the various RNA produced. There are other smaller bodies, all appear to be involved with RNA.

Basically, the nucleolus is the general site of transcription, that is forming RNA from DNA, and modifying the mRNA before it moves onto a ribosome in the cytoplasm to make a protein. During this passage, modifications can be made to this RNA that affects the expression of the DNA. In other words, epigenetics. The transcription of the DNA can be affected by various other molecules which may become attached to the DNA (like methyl groups), or by modifications of histones (next chapter) which can determine whether the DNA will be transcribed or not.

After the RNA has been transcribed, modifications can be made which determine the structure of the protein destined to be formed. The first transcriptions give you the precursor RNA, but this is reorganized to eventually form the mRNA, which is then modified by other types of RNA. By the time the mRNA gets to the ribosome to make a protein, it can be changed in many ways from the original.

Now you can see somewhat what we are talking about in that the DNA has not been changed at all, but the product that results from the transcription of that DNA, (that is if the DNA is even allowed to be transcribed), can be affected by all kinds of other molecules, and these other molecules are changed by the environment.

You may vaguely see where the book is heading. Do not worry, I am going to approach this in several different directions and different examples so that by the end you are going to understand.

INTRODUCTION FO CELL BIOLOGY AND EPIGENETICS

Right now, we must learn a little more lingo and the next chapter will be on DNA. Like Saxon math books, I will go over what you have learned previously as we learn new topics. Like a good language book, I will repeat the lingo over and over as we go along and make longer sentences.

Chapter Four

DNA

We now get to DNA. Most of us know something about this subject. We know that chromosomes are composed of DNA. We know that chromosomes determine our genetic traits, in fact it is our chromosomes that make every animal and plant different from each other. Humans have 46 chromosomes. This is really 22 pairs of chromosomes and one pair of sex chromosomes. We remember that we get 22 chromosomes from each parent to make up those 22 pairs, and a sex chromosome from each parent. Males have one Y and one X, females have XX.

For almost all of us, this has been all we needed to know about DNA our entire lives. I am afraid I am going to teach you a little more. Not enough to be a research scientist, but enough to be able to speak a little lingo and understand what is going on in this field.

First DNA. The stands for deoxyribonucleic acid. Sounds complicated but by the end of the chapter you will be able to draw this molecule, or at least a little bit of it.

DNA is one molecule. Each chromosome has one DNA molecule. We have a basic understanding as to what a molecule is and use this in daily life. Molecules are composed of atoms. We know water is a molecule, as are proteins, fats, sugars, enzymes, and basically our whole body. DNA is the largest biological molecule found in nature. It is one giant molecule made up of a lot of smaller molecules.

How big you may ask. D The average human cell is about 10-40 micrometers. A red blood cell is about 8 micrometers. The largest would be the egg cell, which is about 100 micrometers in diameter, about the size of a human hair. The ovum can often be seen without a microscope, assuming you have good near vision. The typical cell diameter would be about a tenth of the diameter of a hair.

If we compare the volume of a sperm cell with that of the ovum, the sperm is 30 cubic micrometers, one of the smallest cells; while the egg is 4 million cubic micrometers, the largest. I'll do the math for you. The volume of the egg is 100,000 times the volume of the sperm.

The DNA lives in the nucleus of the cell, which is around 10% of the cell volume and has a diameter of 10 micrometers. So, say the cell is about 100 micrometers, the nucleus is about 10 micrometers. All your DNA must be crammed into the nucleus.

INTRODUCTION FO CELL BIOLOGY AND EPIGENETICS

One strand of DNA, which is one molecule, is about two inches long. This is the average as the chromosomes are different sizes thus have different amounts of DNA. Since you have 46 chromosomes, this means if you lined all the DAN up end to end in a row, it would be about seven feet long. This is all crammed into a dot about a tenth of the diameter of a human hair or about 10 microns.

But remember the DNA is composed of atoms which are exceedingly small. Hence, although it is seven feet long, it is only 2 nanometers (one hundred millionth of an inch thick. Hence you would not be able to see it no matter how good your eyesight. The diameter of DNA is about one thousandth the diameter of the nucleus.

A DNA molecule is exceptionally long, but very skinny. Nevertheless, they all must be crammed into the nucleus. As we will see, your body has efficient ways to cram all of these in.

The best way I remember the structure of DNA is to compare it to a ladder. A ladder has rails on either side, and rungs connecting the rails.

The rails are alternating phosphate groups connected to alternating sugar groups. Phosphorus is a mineral like calcium, which combine to form healthy bones. It is easily found in your diet. A phosphate group is a phosphate atom combined with four oxygen atoms. Three single bonds and one double bond, with at least one of the oxygen atoms bonded to another atom. In the case of DNA, one oxygen in the phosphate group is bonded to a carbon atom in the top of a ribose sugar, its downstairs neighbor phosphate group is bonded to a different carbon of the same ribose sugar molecule on the bottom of that molecule. I have the rail of the ladder composed of alternating phosphate-ribose sugar bonds.

The alternating sugar groups are ribose molecules. This means they contain five carbon atoms. Glucose is similar but contains six carbon atoms.

We often draw these molecules in a cyclic formation Ribose has five carbons. It is drawn to look like a pentagon with one of the carbon atoms replaced by oxygen. The fifth carbon atom is bonded to the fourth carbon but sticks out of the ring. We have a nice pentagon with a carbon atom handle sticking out. This carbon handle is called the five prime carbon and attaches to the oxygen atom on the phosphate group which is opposite the double bonded oxygen on the phosphate group. We can call this oxygen atom the bottom of the phosphate group.

Remember, the DNA is composed of two rails of the ladder, and each rail goes in the opposite direction.

This sounds confusing but it is handy to be able to call one direction the 5-prime end, and the other direction the 3-prime end.

The 5- prime carbon handle sticks out of the pentagon, attaches to the 4-prime carbon within the pentagon, and the next atom below in the pentagon is the 3-prime carbon which attaches to the next phosphate group down.

The 5- prime atom attaches to the oxygen in the phosphate group that is opposite the double oxygen bond of that group, the 3 prime atom attaches to an oxygen that is next to the double bonded oxygen of the lower phosphate group. The rails run in opposite directions so if you start at the top end of a DNA string, one side will start with a 5 prime carbon atom, the opposite with a 3- prime carbon atom. Now we can determine directions by saying go toward the 5 prime end or the 3-prime end. We usually depict DNA when we diagram it as the 5-prime on the left heading toward the top.

We have a line of phosphate groups with one oxygen of the group bonded to a ribose on top, and a different oxygen in that same group bonded to a ribose group on the bottom.

We have the rails of the ladder. Now let us look at the rungs. The rungs are composed of what are called base pairs. There are four different nucleobases in DNA. Let us go over some confusing definitions.

Nucleotide is a phosphate group with a five-carbon sugar attached, which is then attached to a nucleobase.

Nucleoside is a nucleobase attached to a five-carbon sugar. In other words, nucleotide without phosphate.

Nucleobase is one of four molecules in DNA. These are cytosine, thymine, adenine, or guanine. These all contain a nitrogen atom.

The rungs of the ladder are composed of two nucleobases bonded together.

Back to the ladder. If I take this ladder with side rails and rungs and split it into two rails, one side of the rung will contain a nucleobase, and the other side will contain a different nucleobase. These nucleobases are usually joined together to make the ladder a single molecule with two bases making up the rungs.

The bases come together is pairs such that if the base on one side of the rung is thymine, the other side will always be adenine. If the adenine is the one on that side, the other side will then be thymine. The same with the other two nucleobases guanine and cytosine. If one side is guanine, the other will always be cytosine and so on.

You can have two cytosines in a row on one side of the ladder, and of course the other side will have two guanines in a row. You can have several in a row if you want. It does appear that a CG pair followed by a GC pair is a favorite occurrence.

We have a ladder with rails made of phosphate and sugar groups, and the rungs made of base pairs. Everything is bonded together to make one giant long molecule.

At this point we need to know the difference between DNA and RNA . The difference is in the five-carbon sugar. DNA means deoxyribonucleic acid. This means the five-carbon sugar contains a hydrogen group at the 2 prime carbon instead of a hydroxyl group which is a hydrogen/oxygen group. So, deoxyribose contains one less oxygen atom than ribose. Deoxy means one less oxygen.

Now a nucleotide of DNA means a phosphate group with a deoxy sugar attached which is then attached to a nucleobase.

A nucleotide of RNA means a phosphate group and a base with a ribose sugar attached.

Sounds like a small change but this makes a big difference. DNA is the repository of genetic information, RNA turns this information into actual structures like protein, fats, and carbohydrates.

The lack of this one oxygen atom per five carbon sugar gives DNA mechanical flexibility and allows it to assume a double helix. This is the ladder twisted around 360 degrees. This also gives DNA the ability to make exceptionally long strands, which RNA does not. RNA is also usually single stranded.

The other difference between DNA and RNA is that RNA uses the nucleobase uracil instead of thymine. In RNA the base pairs are adenine and cytosine just like

DNA, but the other base pair is guanine and uracil, not thymine like DNA.

I am going to talk about RNA in the next chapter, and then we will talk about DNA and RNA together, that is RNA reproducing the genetic information that DNA carries.

I know this sounds complicated and confusing, but you have the ability to understand this information. It seems difficult because it is new lingo to most of us, but like a foreign language, once we start using it in sentences it is much clearer. Like my previous book on Diet and Health, I had to spend several chapters explaining metabolism; but by the end of the book the readers were fluent in that language. So it is which DNA, chromosomes, and epigenetics. You will be fluent by the end of the book.

I still do not think I have impressed you with the length on DNA. The construction is easy with an alternating phosphate group with deoxy ribose sugar forms the rails. The rungs between the rails are formed by two different nucleobases. The entire ladder is twisted around 360 degrees so now we a double helix formation. This occurs every ten feet of the ladder.

    Let us say the ladder is six feet wide and the rungs are one foot apart. I know this is a strange looking ladder, but I must keep the proportions correct. We will have a DNA ladder about 28 thousand miles, or basically around the earth.

    I will return to the ladder in subsequent chapters. We have 26 ladders (chromosomes) in the nucleus, I am giving you the average ladder size as the chromosomes are different lengths. Also, the ladders are quite flexible. Over those 28,000 miles, there are segments where the bases are not connected. There are also segments in which the phosphate groups are not connected, and part of the helix is unwound. This giant ladder is constantly undergoing changes and DNA and RNA are being reproduced or transcribed. More about next chapter. Time to rest your brain a little.

Chapter Five
RNA

Now a little about RNA. I will tell you the basics, but we will revisit RNA several times. Eventually I may tell you about transcription which is how DNA ends up making a protein for your toenail.

But first I must review a little math. My wife usually does not pay any attention to what I write, but I had left the last chapter on my computer, and she happened to look at it. She was probably making sure I was not doing anything crazy like trying to get a real estate license, and she read about the DNA ladder. She did not believe my math example could possibly be correct, so I will briefly go through the math for you.

INTRODUCTION FO CELL BIOLOGY AND EPIGENETICS

Most of us understand scientific notation. It is quite handy. I can write 1000 as 1 X 10^3. We have agreed that 10^0 equals one. If I multiply 10^3 times 10^2, all I have to do is add the exponents, so the result is 10^5. If I divide 10^5 by 10^3, I just subtract 5-3 and get 10^2. Which is 100. Remember that 1 X 10^{-2} is .01. So, 10^3 divided by 10^{-2} results in $10^{3-(-2)}$ which is 10^5. We see 1000/.01 equals 100,000.

The diameter of DNA is 20 X 10^{-10} meters, at least that is what the books say. The distance between base pairs is about 3.4 x 10^{-10}. That is why my ladder looks a little weird because if I make the distance between base pairs to be one foot apart, the width of the ladder must be 20/3.4 equals about 6 feet.

The average chromosome has 150,000,000 base pairs. That means my ladder is 1.5 x 10^8 feet long. To convert that to miles I divided it by 5.280 x 10^3. This gives me 2.84 x 10^4, which is about 28,000 miles. The circumference of the earth is about 25, 000 miles. I am trying to give you a picture of the enormous amount of information in an average DNA molecule. You have 46 of these molecules in the nucleus of practically all the cells.

A long RNA molecule would have a few thousand base pairs, which means on the ladder it would be less than a mile. In real life the length of an average chromosome (one DNA molecule) is about two inches.

I might as well tell you now that there is no stretched out DNA in real life. You cannot really stretch out a chromosome. I told you about histone proteins earlier; they are a group of molecules that wrap the DNA string around like a spool, thought it only wraps around once per histone group. The DNA is wrapped around a bunch of these spools, and the spools themselves coil around each other. When you see pictures of chromosomes, this represents the coiled-up histones arranged in a nice linear configuration as they are preparing to divide and reproduce. More on histones latter. Nevertheless, the ladder image is going to be useful to us. My wife will probably never read the ladder explanation.

    RNA is ribonucleic acid.

    DNA is deoxyribonucleic acid.

The difference is the 2-prime carbon in the pentose sugar group in RNA has a hydroxyl group (OH), and the 2-prime carbon in DNA has a hydrogen atom (H). It is missing the oxygen atom, hence the name deoxy. The rest of RNA is the same as DNA except the complimentary base to adenine in DNA is thymine, whereas in RNA it is uracil. We will visit these later.

    I will review the pentose sugar. This is a pentagon with oxygen replacing carbon at one spot. It then has the 5-prime carbon sticking up like a tootsie roll. This 5-prime carbon combines with the upper phosphate group. The 4 prime carbon is connected to the 5-prime, the 3-prime carbon is connected to the 4-prime carbon and to the lower phosphate group, the 2-prime carbon has (OH) in RNA and (H)in DNA, and the 1-prime carbon is connected to one of the nuclear bases. All three of these groups combined form what is called a nucleotide. A nucleoside is a nucleotide without the phosphate group.

    Both RNA and DNA are nucleic acids. The nuclear bases for nucleic acids are nitrogen containing groups and are cytosine which pairs with guanine (and visa-versa) and adenine which pairs with thymine in DNA, and uracil in RNA.

RNA is almost always single stranded, that is one side of a ladder, while DNA almost always looks like a ladder. RNA is made and changed all the time while DNA is almost always just the same, even after having been duplicated through cell reproduction.

INTRODUCTION FO CELL BIOLOGY AND EPIGENETICS

    I may get to transcription in a while, but most of us already know DNA is split apart and a segment of this DNA is copied by RNA to be transported elsewhere. RNA can then be modified all over the place. It can even double back on itself, bind to itself, and form complex structures which act like proteins. Ribosomes are made of protein and RNA. The RNA dictates which protein the ribosome makes, and the process by which the RNA makes the protein is composed of RNA itself, often in a complex three-dimensional arrangement. This never happens to DNA.

    Epigenetics is the expression of DNA which does not involve any changes in the nuclear base pairs. There are changes in the DNA which can either silence or encourage replication, and these changes are related to the cellular environment. One of the main ways these changes occur is by the manipulation of the RNA which is always undergoing fundamental rearrangement. Your DNA may faithfully produce a piece of RNA, but this piece may look quite different by the time it reaches the ribosome to be made into a protein. It is also regulated along the way to encourage protein manufacturing , or perhaps to stop the manufacturing of the protein altogether, and sometimes to make something different from what it was originally coded to do. What happens to this RNA is a function of the environment, not the DNA.

    RNA comes in several different forms with several different names, and I am going to start on this lingo by listing them. We will see them again later. By the way, DNA does have a couple different forms. When we say DNA, we mean B-DNA There is an A-DNA with different groove sizes, and a Z-DNA formed by methylation of nuclear bases that form a left-handed axis rather than the common right-handed axis. We can ignore these different forms of DNA as

INTRODUCTION FO CELL BIOLOGY AND EPIGENETICS

B-DNA is by far the most common in the cell. We cannot ignore the different RNA.

mRNA (messenger) is the RNA initially formed by the DNA via transcription in which the RNA is copied onto DNA. OK, that is not really true. The first thing formed is pre-mRNA (precursor-mRNA) This must be processed to form the mRNA. It turns out the initial piece of RNA contains regions of nucleotide sequences that do not seem to code for a protein. These regions are called introns. The regions in between the introns which code for a protein are called exons. This also means that within the DNA that was transcribed, there were numerous strings of nucleotides that did not seem to code for anything. Sometimes these segments are called junk DNA.

If we remove the introns, we can then recombine the exon pieces. So, even before the mRNA begins a journey, it has been modified. It is modified even further because when the introns are removed, the exons are sometimes not put back together in the same order. We have changed the coding of the DNA without changing the DNA. This whole process is called splicing. When they are not put back in the same order, we have alternative splicing. In fact, if there are large numbers of introns, you can end up with hundreds of different RNAs by messing up the splicing sequence. This splicing takes place in the nucleus by a small complex of ribonucleoproteins called small nuclear RNP (snRNPs). The complex is called a spliceosome, found in the Cajal bodies. snRNA had about 150 nucleotides.

    We may have only used a few thousand feet of our DNA ladder, and we may have made hundreds of different mRNAs, which may code for thousands of different proteins. This is just in one of our 46 chromosomes.

    The alternative splicing is not random but appears to be under some control. The histones may be a factor, but then what is controlling the histones? It does appear cellular environmental factors affect splicing and the proteins involved in splicing. The protein environment is quite dynamic and small alterations in the environment, like the pH, the electrolyte content of the fluid, small amount of trace elements, or amounts of certain types of proteins whose rate of manufacture is affected by other environmental factors. These are all epigenetic factors. We will soon find out that methyl groups attached to DNA can silence or enhance the transcription of that portion of DNA. The same is probably true of the spliceosomes in that they also contain either silencers or enhancers.

The leftover introns can be processed to form miRNA (micro-RNA) which I will mention later as being involved in epigenetic control over mRNA by preventing that RNA from making proteins.

On with the RNA list. tRNA is transfer RNA. This can read the mRNA to transfer certain amino acids to the ribosome and attach them to the protein that is being coded by the mRNA.

We also have rRNA which is ribosomal RNA. The ribosomes are composed of protein and rRNA which read the incoming mRNA to help the tRNA form the protein. You can have several ribosomes attached to the same length of mRNA at the same time.

Just like we have silencers and enhancers on the DNA, we have RNA that can bind to mRNA to prevent expression. The process by which this occurs in called RNA interference (RNAi) As time has gone on, these RNA molecules seem to have great potential to suppress some gene expression.

There are two types of small RNA molecules called microRNA (miRNA) and small interfering RNA (siRNA) that are primarily responsible for this RNA interference. Remember RNA comes from DNA, and the RNAi is a way in which the DNA can prevent expression of mRNA. Environmental factors are involved in both the expression of the initial pre-RNA, the splicing together of the exons of this pre-RNA, the control of the alternative splicing to get the final form or mRNA, and now the silencing of some of this RNA.

Practically all the cells have the same DNA. Now you are getting an idea that the same DNA can produce many different types of mRNA which can by itself control the expression of other mRNA. The environment of the proteins, DNA, and RNA will affect how this is expressed. This is a dynamic environment and changes all of the time. I am going to investigate how our diet fits into this complex arrangement, hence the book *Epigenetics in Diet and Health*. We are just starting out.

Both microRNA and Small interfering RNA have about 22 nucleotides and bind via complementary sequences to the mRNA; hence are quite specific to the RNA being silenced, and you can have one gene producing RNA that can silence the production of RNA produced by another gene. Like mRNA, you have {pre-miRNA, which also can undergo editing. There is a lot more to tell you about miRNA as it is involved in obesity and diabetes, but that will be a later chapter. We need more basics.

There are lots of different types of RNA and we are fond of giving them all different prefixes. I will do one more before moving on to a different subject, as even I am starting to get them mixed up. Long non-coding RNA or lncRNA is what it sounds. It is an RNA with at least 200 nucleotides which does not code for any protein. These are involved in regulatory functions, just like small and micro-RNA. We arbitrarily choose 200 nucleotides to differentiate the incRNA from the siRNA and miRNA. Up till now you may have gotten the impression that DNA codes for mainly mRNA to make proteins, but it is really the opposite. Most of the RNA coded, at least 4-5 times as much, is for non-coding RNA We have a long DNA strand, really 46 DNA strands, which can code for RNA. Most of the RNA is used to regulate and modify the RNA that we use to make proteins. Environmental factors in the cells modify and regulate the RNA that modifies and regulates the mRNA which came from the pre-mRNA which was modified and regulated from the environment of the cell which came from the DNA which was modified and regulated by other environmental factors.

Remember 97% of our genome is non-coding DNA. Most of it may be regulating the expression of the DNA. The regulation of this regulatory RNA is driven by the cell environment, which is driven by your diet.

This is starting to get complicated and although I am describing what is happening and teaching you some lingo, I understand hardly any of the mechanisms. Do not worry if you don't either, because you won't. We will understand enough to get a better idea of epigenetics and our diet. I am not sure if anyone really understands the regulation of the regulatory RNA coded by the non-coding DNA comprising most of our genome.

List so far:

mRNA: we started here. The DNA strand is unwound from a histone and different enzymes split apart the DNA such that a copy can be made of that stretch of DNA. That copy is mRNA This is coding RNA.

rRNA This is a non-coding RNA which makes up the ribosomes which constructs protein coded by the mRNA.

INTRODUCTION FO CELL BIOLOGY AND EPIGENETICS

tRNA this is transfer RNA that brings the appropriate amino acid to the ribosome to construct the proteins. This is noncoding RNA.

miRNA microRNA is a small strand of ran (22 nucleotides long which is 22 feet in our ladder) this RNA is involved in the regulation of gene expression or epigenetics. These small segments bind to mRNA and prevent certain parts from being processed. The same miRNA can have many target mRNAs. The miRNA can be made from the introns spliced out of pre-mRNA. There also exists pre-miRNA which cand be edited. This is non-coding RNA.

siRNA is small interfering RNA This is about the same size as miRNA, but it is double stranded like DNA but with uracil instead of thymine. It acts very similar to miRNA.

eRNA enhancer RNA These are long noncoding RNA that are transcribed from the enhancer region of a gene. They are promoters of a gene expression.

When most of us learned about DNA, we understood how the DNA was split apart and a template of RNA was formed. We called this mRNA and learned it went to the ribosome where a protein was formed.

We skipped the part where something regulates the histones to unwrap the DNA to start with. We did not know that really it was precursor mRNA that was formed and could be dramatically changed before coding for the protein. We ignored the gauntlet of different RNAs the mRNA had to go through to safely arrive at the ribosome, and the miRNA that could interfere with the tRNA. The more we find out, the more complicated it gets. And now we know everything is affected by the cellular environment which is constantly changing. I may not understand why, but I do know

INTRODUCTION FO CELL BIOLOGY AND EPIGENETICS

your diet is a major factor in controlling the cellular environment.

Chapter Six
Chromosomes and Genes

The first part of this book is to review what many of us knew and have now forgotten. Let me remind you about chromosomes. By now we recall that chromosomes contain our genetic information, and each chromosome is a long molecule of DNA. Humans have 46 total chromosomes in each cell. These 23 chromosomes are arranged in pairs, so we have 23 pairs. As we all know from school or watching some show on TV, we get one of these pairs from the male and one from the female when the egg and sperm combine. The egg has 23 chromosomes, the sperm 23, and the zygote , or fertilized egg has 46.

You also recall something about genes. Genes are segments of chromosomes that code for certain biological traits. These traits usually require that a protein, or several different proteins are produced.

We have a segment of DNA that codes for the production of a protein. This is done by unzipping the base pairs in this segment of DNA and making a complimentary RNA segment of the exposed bases on one side of the zip. I told you earlier which base pairs match with which, and that RNA uses uracil instead of thymine. We also know that this RNA is really pre-mRNA and may undergo alternative splicing which not only removes the introns (non-coding RNA), but also may recombine the remaining exons in a different order than that which they were originally copied. Hence, we can get one strand of pre-mRNA to code for many different proteins.

Also recall we have pairs of these chromosomes, such that the sister to this chromosome may be slightly different, although the location of the gene is the same on both chromosomes. We call these two, maybe slightly different genes, alleles. An allele is then two different forms of the same gene. I said two, but really there can be more than two different forms. The genes are still located in the same place on each of the paired chromosomes.

Humans have about 25,000 different genes located on the chromosomes. These vary in size up to a couple million base pairs. That still does not take up much of the room available as remember, we have 23 chromosomes, and the average length is 150,000,00 base pairs. I know we really have 46 chromosomes, but each pair looks alike as far as gene locations.

I said we have around 25,000 genes. These vary in length from 25,ooo base pairs to up to two million. Even then, this takes up only 1-2% of our genome. Most of our DNA is not composed of genes. We call this noncoding DNA, but that is not really correct. This DNA has the capacity to code for all kinds of things, we have just not recognized for what. We already know about the various RNA that is being formed and now realize that this RNA may control the expression of genes. In other words, this is one of the mechanisms by which epigenetic changes occur.

It ends up that a fair portion of this non gene DNA may be of viral origin. Segments of viral DNA appear in our genome and these segments can actually move around by inserting and copying themselves in other segments of the chromosome, or even in other chromosomes. Even these viral segments are subject to epigenetic controls.

These viral segments are known as endogenous retroviruses and can make up 8% of the genome.

I may talk more about genetics later, but first I find confusion about what is a gene. Let us use eye color. We can find an area of a chromosome that codes for genes that seem to control eye color. It is quite handy to know which chromosome and where on the chromosomes the genes reside. We were able to find this area because we examined phenotypes. A phenotype is an observable characteristic. It is the expression of the DNA.

It is true that once we identified this area, we could then determine the base pairs and perhaps even identify different enzymes involved. We are just looking at this particular trait. The cell that contains melanin has all kinds of other processes going on in that cell with maybe a thousand different enzymes whose DNA may be on many different chromosomes. This cell still must produce energy and use glucose which requires transcription for enzymes that are used in many other cells. When we say,

"Here is the gene that controls eye color", we must realize this is only a small part of the expression of the total DNA of that cell.

Well, how about that. We have circled back around to epigenetics, the expression of your DNA. We have the eye color gene and have identified the DNA involved, and now have solved the eye color situation. Wait a minute. If you have been paying any attention, you know that the expression of the DNA is modified by all kinds of environmental factors. We know about alternate splicing and how genes may code for certain mRNA, but that does not mean we know what the mRNA will look like when it finally gets expressed.

Genes are quite handy in our understanding of genetics and provide a way to locate certain areas of chromosomes. Using our ladder, we have DNA going around the world, and the gene we want occupying a few miles of it. It is nice to be able to narrow the location down a bit. It's like knowing the address of one house around the world. If we were just checking each house randomly, it would take quite a while to find the house you were looking for.

We will remember that this area which codes for our brown eyes by translating the DNA into RNA may not change, but the expression may. Maybe depending on the environment. Your eyes may get browner over time. The DNA did not change, but you have undergone epigenetic changes.

Now back to chromosomes. I have mentioned this before and now is the time to talk more about histones. Your DNA is not present in the nucleus of the cell in a linear condition. It just will not fit. Instead, it is complexed with proteins, and those proteins are called histones. Recall that the linear chromosomes are wrapped around these histone proteins such that the giant DNA molecule is 40,000 to 50,000 times smaller than if it were stretched out. The segments of DNA are unable to code for RNA unless they are unwrapped from these histones.

The histones exist as a group of eight histone proteins. There are four major types of histone proteins and eight are combined to form the histone core around which the DNA wraps itself. A piece of DNA wrapped around a histone is called a nucleosome. This nucleosome is composed of about 146 base pairs, then there is a gap of approximately 50 base pairs of DNA, till the next nucleosome. There is a histone protein that binds the DNA at the entry and exit sites of the nucleosome, hence the DNA is somewhat fixed in place. This allows this string of beads to be wound around to form different string configurations.

Each histone is formed by two copies of the four core histones. There are segments of proteins which extend out of the cores called histone tails. These histone tails bind to various regions of the DNA and with other nucleosomes. If we remove the histone tails, the DNA of the histone has increased accessibility and hence is more active to form mRNA. It therefore appears that the histone tails may be a major factor in controlling the epigenetic expression of DNA by regulating the ability of that DNA to be accessible. For transcription.

I feel obligated to mention James Bonner and Ru Chih Chow Huang, who in the late 1960s showed that isolated chromatin (DNA wrapped around histones) would not support RNA transcription unless you unwrapped the histones. This was a leap forward and the research was done when it was immensely difficult to perform.

Now we know we need histones to condense the DNA into the nucleus. We know that the DNA must be unwound from the histones to make RNA. We know that histone tails interact with the DNA and other histones to somehow control expression of DNA by allowing the DNA to be transcribed into RNA.

    The histone proteins are of course formed by transcription of histone DNA. These proteins then undergo modifications, mainly of the tails, that affect how these histones interact with DNA and other histones. I will go into details later, but the main modifications of these histones involve adding a methyl (CH_4) group which is methylation, or an acetyl group (C_2H_3O) which is acetylation. This is how epigenetics works through histones, now let us see how it works through changing the expression of DNA.

Chapter Seven
Methylation and Acetylation

To understand the role of methylation of DNA, we must understand the concept of CpG islands. First what are we talking about. I hope you still remember that C stands for cytosine, one of the nucleobases in DNA, and G stands for guanine. These are base pairs and represent one rung of the DNA ladder. If the next rung (going in the 5' to 3' direction is a Guanine to Cytosine base pair, this combination is called a CpG site.

    Recall our ladder. The rungs of the ladder are two base pairs connected by hydrogen bonds. The sides of the ladder (the rails) are connected together by phosphate to sugar bonds. This is the backbone of the ladder. One rail starts out at the 5' position, the opposite side starts at the 3' end. The 5' end is a phosphate group, the 3' end is a hydroxyl group.

Everyone agreed with this system, so we know which direction we are going on the rails. One rail goes 3" to 5', the other side the opposite.

To avoid confusion, a CG pair is just a rung of the ladder containing the CG base pair, A CpG site is two rungs of the ladder, the first with a CG base pair, the next with a GC base pair. These two rungs are connected by a p (phosphate) at the rails; hence this is described as a CpG site. If you have a bunch of these CpG sites in a row, you have what is called CpG islands.

A methyl group can be added to the cytosines of the CpG by the enzyme DNA methyltransferase. It turns out that about 75% of these CpG cytosines are methylated.

We would expect based on statistics that a CpG dinucleotide (a CG pair followed by a GC pair) would occur about 4% of the time. Ends up in the human genome we see it less than 1% of the time. Sometimes the methylated cytosine in the CpG undergoes spontaneous removal of a nitrogen group (deamination) which turns the methylated cytosine into thymine, a different base. Now you have a mismatched GT base pair which your repair enzymes may resolve to AT instead of back to GC.

The Cytosine to Thymine spontaneous transformation can occur at unmethylated sites, but it is ten times higher at the methylated sites.

So we have fewer CpG sites than expected, but we also have CpG islands which are regions with a high frequency of CpG sites.

INTRODUCTION FO CELL BIOLOGY AND EPIGENETICS

By now you may be asking "why do we care about the CpG sites"? There are promoter regions in DNA. This is a sequence of DNA to which proteins bind to initiate transcription. The transcription of DNA into mRNA doesn't just start anywhere and these regions are the starting points. CpG islands, about a couple thousand base pairs in length, are associated with these promoter regions. These islands contain many more CpG groups than would be expected. Multiple methylated CpG site in the promoter region silences the expression of the following gene. In other words, that gene (section of DNA) is not expressed or transcribed.

I should clarify. The CpG islands are not a continuous line of CpG base pairs, but a high frequency of them.

In the body of the gene, that is the coding part that we are copying to make mRNA or something else, the methylated cytosines present in CpG sites may enhance the expression of the gene. as opposed to suppressing it.

Methylation was the key to our understanding of how epigenetics works. Before we knew much about epigenetics, we did know that one of the X chromosomes was inactivated in the female somatic cells such that a Barr body was formed, a condensation of an X chromosome. We knew that this chromosome was inactive but not the mechanism.(we now believe that these Barr bodies are not totally inactive and may code for RNA) Support was demonstrated for the idea that methylation of cytosine was the mechanism by which this was accomplished with the use of 5-azacytidine, a nucleoside analogue. When this was incorporated into DNA instead of cytosine, DNA methyl transferase (the enzyme that attaches a methyl group to cytosine) removed the methyl group from 5 methyl cytosine and reactivated the silenced X chromosome as well as other silenced genes. This also revealed that some genes that were abnormal and we thought had mutations were really on silenced and could be reactivated. Now we know this is an extensive mechanism used in epigenetics.

Let me briefly mention bisulfate sequencing. Treating DNA with bisulfate before sequencing (figuring out the order of nucleotides) to determine the methylation pattern was markedly assisted as it converts cytosine to uracil but leaves 5-methycytosine unaffected Now you can figure out the extent of methylation in a sequence of DNA.

Recall epigenetics is the expression of DNA. The cellular environment drives varied expression of this DNA. The mechanisms as to how this is accomplished is often through the methylation of either histones or cytosine bases. We have discovered several ways this is accomplished, but why it happened is still too complex. Your cellular environment is mainly controlled by what you eat, in other words your diet. It also includes absorption through your lungs, skin and even radiation effects that can change your internal environment.

I told you at the beginning this is a series of books titled *Epigenetics in Diet and Health.* I have already written the series *Diet and Health.* In it you found out that if you eat a lot of carbs, you get fat. I reviewed some biochemistry as to how this is accomplished but did not mention at all why it happens. We can now say that this is an epigenetic change and begin to see how this is related to the expression of your DNA. Although we may be better at describing what is happening, we do not know why it is happening other than saying high glucose somehow changes the cellular environment and expression of our DNA. I don't have to know how it happens, just tell you to eat better.

One of the basic mechanisms is methylation, often cytosine. This can have different effects depending on where the cytosine is located on the DNA. Last chapter I talked about histones, primarily as to their function in storing DNA and how there is no transcription unless that DNA strand is unraveled from the histone. The histone has its own DNA gene which has a promoter and may be affected by CpG islands, both to initiate the transcription and modify some DNA in the body of the histone protein. We now know the action of the histones can be modified post transcription.

The acetyl groups I talked about affect the tails of the histones. The acetyl modification of the tail may neutralize some of the charges on the proteins and hence loosen the DNA from the histone which allows transcription. This is a post transcription effect. This is another mechanism by which epigenetic changes are produced. The histone tails undergo several other types of modification, but methyl and acetyl appear to be the main ones.

I'm giving you the basics so you can learn the lingo. I don't really need to know any of this to give you a proper diet, but we will learn how the diet affects what is happening at the DNA level. We still don't know all the feedback loops and why this happens, but in the next book I will look at the practical applications. Now we have a few more basics.

In ends up that the hypermethylation of promoter regions which silences genes is an important factor in cancers. We may think of cancer as a mutation which prevents expression of a gene, but hypermethylation of the promoter regions causes silencing of a gene ten times more frequently than mutations.

A mutation could cause a portion of the DNA to code for an abnormality in the gene that could present itself as cancer, but it appears a major cause of cancer may be the lack of expression of the DNA repair genes.

Methylation of cytosine may be a permanent effect in some cells. This is best seen in the initial differentiation of stem cells into cells that do not change. Your heart cells do not change into liver cells. That part of the epigenetic change is permanent and some of that cell DNA will never be expressed. These are referred to as epigenetic marks. At the same time, methylation of cytosine is being reversed all the time in cells. The cells are constantly adapting to their environment and DNA expression is constantly changing. This is part of the reason I am writing all these books to start with. A proper diet may not only keep you healthy, but also may be able to reverse some of the changes you have induced by a poor diet. I am not saying diet will cure cancer, but it may be able to change some of the epigenetic changes that induced it.

A couple chapters ago we talked about microRNA (miRNA) which can bind to portions of mRNA and prevent expression. We now recognized that in certain cancers the promoter region in the DNA that is coding for these miRNAs is hypermethylated. This means these miRNAs are being suppressed. That means that those miRNAs are not available to silence mRNA which means that you are allowing increased expression of a lot of other genes which seems to lead to cancers. I just told you that the lack of suppression is much more commonly caused by hypermethylation than by mutation. Hypermethylation is an epigenetic change. You now know that epigenetic changes are induced by the environment of the cell.

INTRODUCTION FO CELL BIOLOGY AND EPIGENETICS

If I told not eating enough fiber increased your risk for colon cancer, would you then think that the fiber was somehow keeping a mutation from happening in the colon cell. Or, after reading *Diet and Health*, you would you know that fiber is carbohydrate for which we do not have the enzymes to digest, but which the gut bacteria in the colon do have. As a result of this, alcohols as well as other chemicals are released into the colon and used by the colonocytes. As you would expect, this affects the internal environment of those cells. This then causes a different epigenetic environment as opposed to those who don't eat much fiber. This may then affect the methylation status of different promoter regions in the colon cell DNA such that there is not hypermethylation of certain promoter sites in the DNA coding for certain miRNA. This will affect the miRNA environment and the normal suppression of various genes or gene products that may lead to cancer may not occur as much. In other words, maybe no mutations are involved, but rather just a different diet.

This is just an example, and the actual process of cancer development is much more complicated, so much so that we cannot completely understand it. I am trying to get you to think a little differently. You do have a great deal of control over your diet. Epigenetics is a major factor in health and cancer, and diet is the controller of your intracellular environment for the most part. You can't just eat right for a weekend; you must develop the correct lifetime maintenance diet for yourself.

By the way, I forgot to mention DNA repair genes. You undergo DNA damage all the time; it is a normal part of cell life. You have an abundance of DNA repair genes that fix this damaged DNA You can imagine that if you had hypermethylation of the CpG islands in the promoter DNA of these genes and they were silenced that this would be a bad thing. In fact, it is. We do believe DNA damage may be the underlying cause of cancer, but the lack of repair of this DNA and the excess expression of other genes due to epigenetic changes may be the reason one person gets cancer and another doesn't, even though everyone is getting DNA damage throughout their life.

    At this point I need to add some extra information. If you read the above paragraph and think about it, you may recall something called the BRCA1 gene This stands for BReast CAncer gene. Now before you start thinking this is a gene that causes cancer, read on a little.

    Your body was designed to live a very long time. This means you have many systems designed to act as maintenance systems. You have autophagy, which is a cellular process that occurs in cells with a nucleus which identifies abnormal structures in the cell, including DNA, RNA, any of the cell structures I have talked about, and encloses these structures in a vacuole and attaches various chemicals which breaks this structure down into its components to be used again. It uses these elements for energy, or to make other things. Your cell can reproduce any structure in the cell, including duplicating the entire cell.

You cell also has a system that ensures the DNA is reproduced exactly. There are usually several genes which code for elements that ensures this. This makes sense has you DNA is being transcribed or reproduced millions of times a day in your body. After seventy years that's billions of times. It is essential that these reproductions are exact.

At the same time , your cells are exposed to many different chemicals in the environment. Thes can damage your DNA, such that it does not work correctly, or can influence the expression of the DNA, which is epigenetics. Your body is quite active at the cellular level.

BRCA genes code for the proteins involved in insuring the DNA is repaired if any damage occurs. This gene itself contains various mutations which make parts of this repair process fail. The BRCA-1 and BRCA-2 are two identified mutations in this gene that prevents repair of damaged DNA and hence increases the chance of breast cancer, and several other cancers, developing.

Cancer develops when you have abnormal DNA. This could result from a continuous exposure to various environmental elements, dysfunction of the repairs processes (and usually several must go wrong to get cancer), or a genetic factor such as BRCA.

There is much information on testing for BRCA and what to do with these results. There are just as many males with the BRCA genes as there are females, and the males have increased incidence of some cancers. In females, this abnormal gene significantly increases breast and ovarian cancer,

If you grandmother had the gen, that means about half of her offspring, that is your mother may have it, and about half of her offspring may have it. The same thing applies if it was your grandfather is the one who had it.

Now it doesn't sound so crazy when we ask about your grandparent's health.

INTRODUCTION FO CELL BIOLOGY AND EPIGENETICS

Virus

Now we get to talk a little about viruses. This is convenient as now all we hear about are viruses. It is also going to be much easier as the virus uses all the things we have talked about.

A virus does not have any of the machinery that the cell has. It is basically just a piece of DNA or RNA, a receptacle for these, and some type of protein vehicle that allow access to the cell. Once in the cell it can then take over.

I explained the size of DNA by making a ladder that went around the world. I will need a different example for a virus.

Let's imagine a cell the size of a woman's basketball. A virus would be the equivalent of a mustard seed on the surface of this basketball. We are now dealing in a whole new realm.

Brownian motion is the continuous erratic random motion of very small particles as a result of the bombardment of these particles.

The cells in your body are slightly affected by this phenomenon, and the smaller the particle, the more it is affected.

I am going to use the Covid virus as an example to explain viruses. By now all of you have seen a picture of this virion. It is a sphere with projections around this sphere, around forty projections.

These projections are called spike proteins. Each projection is really three spike proteins curled around each other.

If you have the virion next to the basketball, the virion is about the size of a mustard seed. The spike protein is a fourth of the size of the virion.

Now the covid virion is an RNA virus. There are some viruses that are DNA viruses. This segment of RNA can code for 29 proteins. As you can see, this is not very many compared to the human DNA. For the structure of the virus, there are only four proteins. The rest of the proteins are going to be used once the virus gets inside. If we use the previous example I gave you of the DNA ladder, this is about 5 miles worth of ladder.

A cell in your body has the ability to reproduce itself. That means it has the machinery and the instructions from the DNA to make every little thing in the cell.

The virus has no ability to make anything. Every virus has been reproduced by a cell somewhere. For a virus to survive, it must enter a cell somewhere and convince that cell to begin making more viruses using the DNA or the RNA that the virus bought with them.

INTRODUCTION FO CELL BIOLOGY AND EPIGENETICS

The mustard seed is much smaller than the basketball, yet somehow it must take over control of the cell in order to reproduce. It barely has any RNA (or DNA), yet it survives.

You may not believe a mustard seed can take over a basketball, but if you plant a mustard seed in the ground it can grow to be as large as a basketball.

Viruses have various ways to enter the cells. The cell membrane is quite complex, and things are entering and leaving all the time. These almost always need to be transported through the cell membrane, generally into some type of cystic structure.

Things are bumping into the cells all the time. Brownian motion encourages this as well as the fluid in which the cell resides. Viruses are so small that even the very small electric forces on the surface of the cells influences the actions of viruses.

Let me continue using the covid virus as an example. You saw those stalks on the surface of the virion, this is the way the covid virus gets its RNA into the cell. The ends of the stalks have an area which can react is one of the receptors on the cell membrane. The cell membrane has hundreds of receptors. We want certain things in the cell like various enzymes or proteins or fatty acids or insulin or glucose. There are lots of things going into and out of this membrane all the time. The membrane is the barrier, and the various receptors are gates to this barrier.

The receptors can recognize a particular element and facilitate entry to the cell. Your membrane is quite protective as to what it lets in.

As I said before, things are bumping into the cell membrane constantly, and most of the time in order to get into the cell they must activate a receptor of some kind.

INTRODUCTION FO CELL BIOLOGY AND EPIGENETICS

These receptors are very small. The covid virion stalk proteins have a small area at the tip of the stalk which must come into contact with an even smaller receptor on the cell membrane in order to activate certain enzymes in both the covid virion and the cell membrane. The mustard seed has a stalk with is on fourth the size of the seed and the area on the stalk that needs to encounter the receptor is about one fifth the size of the stalk protein, and the receptor is small that this area. You can see it may not be that easy for a virion to infect the cell.

Once the stalk does encounter the receptor, changes occur in the stalk such that it bends over to allow the virus to come into direct contact with the cell membrane. This in turn activates other enzymes such that the virion can be enveloped by the cell or just insert the RNA into the cell.

Your body knows what to do with RNA, and it is transported to a ribosome, just like all the other RNA in the cytoplasm. In this case, once the proteins in the viral genome are transcribed, they take action to take over the cell.

In real life, the stalk protein is about thirty glucose molecules long. You may wonder how anyone can ever get infected with all these processes going on to even enable to stalk to find and connect with a receptor. The answer is that you have lots of virions. At the height of an infection your body produces 1-10 billion virions with a single cell making about one million a day.

At this point you may be asking yourself "why in the world do the cell membrane have a rector for covid to tart with"? Well, it doesn't. For covid, the receptor interacts with the same receptor for the angiotensin converting enzyme. This enzyme helps regulate the renin-angiotensin-aldosterone system.

INTRODUCTION FO CELL BIOLOGY AND EPIGENETICS

Covid is just hijacking this receptor to get into the cell. Other viruses may sneak in through other receptors. The ACE2 receptor is present in epithelium in the nose, mouth, and lungs. You inhale covid virions, it gets into the mucosal layer, it gets to the cell, and finally invades the cell. Once the cell is infected it begins making a bunch of virions which then spread to cells

The virus is the size of a mustard seed, a bacterium is about ten times as large.

CHAPTER 8

EPIGENETICS

I originally was going to put a chapter on genetics here. As time passed and I continued to think on these topics, I realized genetics has very little to do with my goal: which is to prevent Type 2 diabetes.

I have concluded T2DM is a dietary disease, not a genetic disease. You develop an abnormal metabolism, and this is manifested by obesity. You progress and eventually get elevated insulin levels. You then get elevated glucose levels and reach he definition of diabetes, which is elevated glucose. This happens over a period of years. You eventually may get low insulin levels, but that doesn't make any difference. The definition of diabetes is high glucose, regardless of the insulin level.

If we look at family portraits, we see some in which everyone appears to be fat. You would logically assume that there must be an inherited mutation that runs in this family. Many have looked for chromosome aberrations that let us say if you have this mutation, you will be obese. Other than quite rate mutations, this does not seem to exist. Now we have 40% of the world obese. Is this an epidemic of mutations or something else? I'll give you the answer, it is something else.

You know a little about epigenetics. Throughout our life our epigenome changes. In fact, it is constantly changing. I told you it appears some changes are permanent. We know that some epigenetic marks can be passed on to the next generation; but strange as it sounds, none of this is genetic. We cannot biopsy one of your early undifferentiated cells (blastomeres), look at the chromosomes, and predict if this person will be fat. I have already written a book on why you get fat. The short version is that it is your diet. Now I am trying to tell you how it happened in an attempt to get you to change your diet to one that does not predispose you to T2DM. The diet today is not the same as the diet from the last 5000 years.

    If we start the epigenetic story from the beginning, we must start before you were born. In fact, before you were conceived. Your mother's eggs (oocytes) in her ovaries were grown while your mother was in your grandmother's womb. While she was a fetus several million oocytes were created. By the time your mother was born, this number had dropped to less than a million. Remember the oocytes to not replicate. The oocytes in your mother's ovaries are the same ones that were created when she was in her mother's womb. Oocytes are perhaps the longest living cells in a female's body. Even when your mother is a grandmother, there will still be a few oocytes present in her ovary. They will be older than she is.

We know epigenetic changes are related to cellular environment which is determined by diet among other factors. Diet is a broad term. We are ingesting many chemicals in our diet without knowing it, by inhalation, skin absorption, drinking water, and whatever chemicals are on the things we eat. These factors cause epigenetic changes throughout your life, often manifested by the methylation of the CpG sites. As we age some of these CpG islands become over methylated, some undermethylated.

We get two chances to erase these methylations. When the germ cells become haploid at the time of meiosis, and when the sperm and egg combine at the time of fertilization. The sperm involved in your conception are about three months old.

The eggs are about thirty years old. We now can demonstrate some epigenetic effects related to the brief cellular environmental exposure of the sperm. Of course, the eggs have been exposed to the grandmother's and mother's environment. The significant exposure is when the stem cells were creating the germ cells which occurs during the first twelve weeks of gestation.

Your mother is conceived with your grandfather's 3-month-old sperm and your grandmother's 30-year-old egg. This egg has been exposed to epigenetic factors in your grandmother's diet. When fertilization took place, the epigenetic changes were erased, but wait a minute, not all of them were erased. Some of these epigenetic marks were continued in your mothers eggs. Your mother's eggs were then formed while she was in your grandmother's womb and the diet of your grandmother while pregnant appears to have a significant effect on these eggs. You come along and are conceived with your mother's thirty-year-old eggs which may still contain some of your grandmother's epigenetic marks, and your father's three-month-old sperm. Now you are pregnant.

This has all happened without any change in the DNA structure. It does appear the epigenetic marks are not permanent and may therefore change through the generations, unlike the DNA structure. They may or may not get erased during germ cell formation or fertilization.

Wait a minute, Kelly. Are you telling me I am fat because my grandmother was fat? Epigenetic changes are not mutations. They change the expression of the genes. The genes do not change their DNA, just their expression. But yes, if you grandmother and mother are fat, you have an increased chance of being fat. You may have a predisposition, but it is not a given that you will be fat. If both are fat, it probably is because they did not eat a good diet. Your mothers diet through most of the early part of her life was what your grandmother provided. If it was a poor diet, she had a good chance of getting fat. Your diet for the early part of your life was provided by your mother, who most likely learned about diet from her mother. If this was a poor diet, you had a good chance of getting fat.

    I say a chance because we know many epigenetic changes can be reversed, especially early in life. Nobody has genes that make them obese. They may make you husky, taller, more muscular, bigger, or skinnier; but your genes do not make you obese. Epigenetic changes will make you obese and give you T2DM, but these are driven by your diet. You can change that. You can't change your genes. Epigenetic changes may give you a propensity to be fat, but your diet made you fat.

INTRODUCTION FO CELL BIOLOGY AND EPIGENETICS

I am going to make you think a little more. If recall earlier in the book I mentioned mitochondrial DNA. This is circular DNA found in an organelle in the cytoplasm, not in the nucleus. This DNA is from the egg, not sperm. The egg is about 10,000 times the size of the sperm. The sperm does not contain mitochondria, hence all the mitochondria in the zygote come from the egg. That means your mitochondrial DNA comes only from your mother. When you look at mitochondrial DNA (mtDNA) in mature oocytes, you see a lot of copies of DNA. Like your normal DNA, this DNA also undergoes epigenetic changes with methylation at CG sites. The mtDNA codes for only a few of the thousands of genes required for their function. The other genes come from your regular DNA.

This mtDNA undergoes the same processes as nuclear DNA with histone formation and methylation of CpG sites. It appears these epigenetic changes occur in early embryo development. The difference is that when the sperm and egg combine their chromatin and most epigenetic changes are erased, the mtDNA does not undergo erasure. Remember this DNA was in the oocyte that had been in your mother for thirty years and may have undergone epigenetic changes related to the cellular environment. Now you get these epigenetic marks in the mitochondria.

Mitochondria are involved in energy production in the cells of the body. Although the other epigenetic marks may have been erased, these may not have been. If they have had long term exposure to higher-than-normal glucose levels, it would not be surprising if energy metabolism in all the cells may be abnormal and contribute to obesity. Remember, these cells have been exposed both to your grandmother's and mother's diet.

We will talk a little more about this early journey. Most of us have an idea about fertilization. A sperm enters the oocyte, and they combine to form a complete chromosomal package with 23 pairs of chromosomes. It appears that now is when many of the epigenetic marks are erased. The zygote then undergoes cell division without growing. This is called cleavage.

    The zygote divides till there are about 16 cells and forms a blastocyst. At this stage the cells are totipotent, that is able to turn into all the different cell types. At this stage you could also remove one of these cells and check the chromosomes without affecting the morula. The cell will divide a little more, form a blastocyst, and implant into the endometrium. Before this can occur, the cells must begin to differentiate into the ectoderm, mesoderm, and endoderm. These are not totipotential cells but can turn into many different cell types. They cannot turn back into blastomeres. Of course, we can characterize this as an epigenetic process. The cell DNA is the same, but the cells are now different. They are now pluripotent. Eventually all the different cell types in your body are formed.

We don't know why this happens. Like other epigenetic changes, I assume the cellular environment drives this process, but maybe not. When the embryo is growing, we know the environment affects the cells. If you have an elevated glucose environment during the first trimester when the eggs are forming, I believe this may have an epigenetic effect on the egg and eventually will affect the progeny. Again, the chromosomes are the same, but the expression may be different. All of these changes may not be erased during fertilization, especially the mtDNA epigenetic changes.

When I mention the cellular environment, I am including changes in the environment caused by neighboring cells. The cells in your body communicate with each other. This is undoubtably occurring during early embryogenesis when your organs are forming.

I have only introduced you to epigenetics and now you can see how incredibly complex the process is. We may be able to determine some of the enzymes or mechanisms, but we recognize that there is much more to it than we understand.

I am interested in your diet. By now you know that this exerts an influence on how your DNA is expressed, and hence your health. I can derive a lot of this influence by just studying the history of diet and food. I started with how the modern western diet is making everyone in the world fatter. I concluded that this is an epigenetic effect, not a mutation of the chromosomes. I also conclude that your diet has a great influence on your health by the same mechanisms.

In the end, I have given you a guideline for diet that may lead you to your best chance for health.

I have already written the next book in this series entitled *Fat Newborns, Infants, and Kids* in which I will go into more detail about epigenetic changes and give suggestions as to how to stop obesity. My goal is to prevent T2DM. To do that I must get you to eat a proper diet. To do that I must teach you about diet so that you will be more likely to do it. If I want to stop obesity, it appears I must start with the mother's womb.

The third book will be about the gut biome. It's importance to good health is rapidly being realized, and diet drives the gut biome. You may think your diet is what you eat, but it is mainly what you absorb. The gut biome has significant input as to what is absorbed by the intestine. It also modifies almost everything you eat such that you are absorbing altered biological products, not necessarily everything you put in your mouth. If you start looking at the ingredients of processed food, you will see you are eating many chemicals that have never been eaten for most of human history.

You may be eating aspartame thinking it has no calories, but would you be surprised if I told you epigenetic changes in the gut biome may be causing conversion of this artificial sweetener into caloric intake?

WHO has now agreed that what we figured out years ago is true. Artificial sweeteners do not help you lose weight. You may have noticed that the term "diet" in food is slowly being replaced by "zero sugar" food.

I have a separate book on artificial sweeteners. **Allulose and Other Sweeteners.**

CHAPTER 9
DIET AND HEALTH

As I told you before, my goal is to prevent T2DM through a proper diet. In my books I call this a maintenance diet. This is different from a fat losing diet, although you may lose weight on it depending on how bad your diet is now. There are a couple different kinds of maintenance diets.

Because this is my goal, I am going to add a brief review of this diet in the next few pages. I usually include something like this in all my books and will in this one.

The book *Diet and Health* is composed of five smaller books:

Diabetes/Prediabetes/Obesity Management, Prevention, Treatment

INTRODUCTION FO CELL BIOLOGY AND EPIGENETICS

This reviews how you got obesity and diabetes to start with, and what to do about it.

The Ketogenic Diet for Beginners The science behind your diet and why you get fat.

I believe that for most this diet is the best fat losing diet. I do not recommend this for children. It may be appropriate for some obese adolescents. It is appropriate for most adults. This is not a maintenance diet. It is a temporary diet to use till you lose the appropriate amount of fat, then you must switch to a maintenance diet. This diet is not for long term usage as it is not balanced, but the small risk of the diet is worth not having the large risks of obesity related illness if you do not lose fat.

Fasting and Autophagy for the Common Man

I do not advise fasting for children in this book. Remember, not eating 12 hours between the last meal of the day and the first of the next day is not fasting. It is historically normal, and we are designed to do this. Longer fasting is not for children but may be useful for the health of adults. I also discuss hunger; the reason the low-calorie diets fail.

Maintenance Diet for the Modern Man

I go over the various maintenance diets and why you should eat this way. Everyone does not have the same one. Children have the same one as their parents for the most part.

Bread in the Modern Diet

In the written history over the last 5000 years there is a special place for bread. I tell you what bread is and why it is special. Now, modern bread is a major factor in the induction of insulin resistance secondary to wheat processing. You used to be able to survive on bread alone, not now.

I did not discuss food supplements in any of these books. In *Fat Newborns Infants, and Kids* I do advise prenatal vitamins and omega 3 supplements for pregnant women. I also recommend one of the maintenance diets. Pregnancy and breast feeding is a special time diet wise for women. For most of mankind's history we did not take food supplements. That is not to say we did not realize some foods seemed to ameliorate certain disease, or that some diets led to better health, but I am talking about extra vitamins and supplements we see in the health food store.

I do not usually recommend supplements for normal people, but that may change. The food we eat is not the same as that eaten historically. Micronutrients may have changed, the genetics may have changed, especially

GMO, and the nutritional content has changed. I advised omega 3 fatty acids in pregnancy to change the 6:3 ratio. I hope I can do that in normal people by decreasing omega 6 food and increasing omega 3 food, but I am not sure. I am awaiting further information on this subject before giving you advice. That does not mean I might not do this on my own or advise those who have some sort of autoimmune disease such as rheumatoid arthritis to include this in their diet.

The difference in the various maintenance diets is related to carbohydrate intake. Almost everyone has heard of the Mediterranean diet. This divides your food intake into equal portions, calorie wise, of fats, protein, and carbohydrates. I agree with this somewhat and go into much more detail as to which fats, protein, and carbohydrate to eat. In general, I advise a little less carbohydrate intake in some people. My overall goal is to prevent T2DM and maintain good health.

I would like us to return to the normal pattern of eating. First that means the 12 hours of no caloric intake between the last meal of the day and the first. After the age of somewhere between 4 and 6, everyone should be able to do this. Not eating means no caloric intake. If you eat a late dinner, just eat a late breakfast. Metabolically speaking, almost everyone should be able to do this.

The historical normal pattern of eating is to eat when you are hungry and don't eat when you are not. This worked great for most people when they were young. Nobody used to eat after sundown. Now we have artificial light 24 hours a day and eat around the clock. Once we ate twice a day. No lunch. We developed artificial lighting and thus extended the workday, and the play day. A few hundred years ago lunch became the norm. Now eating more than three times a day is the norm. We invented TV and food commercials, as well as the refrigerator and now eating many times a day is the norm. Just one bonbon spikes your insulin. Every time you eat even a bite you get a bump. Eat when you are hungry and don't when you are not.

Children and teenagers need snacks. I discuss this in *Maintenance Diet for the Modern Man.*

Although the historical diet was probably high carb, we cannot do that anymore because the food has changed, mainly through processing, such that it gives us more rapid absorption of glucose. The maintenance diet will be lower carb. This level can drop depending on where you are with insulin resistance.

Here is a brief review of the Maintenance diet.

Decrease soy dramatically. Maybe not zero, as that would be somewhat difficult, but we need to lower omega 6.

Decrease high fructose corn syrup to zero. No one ate any 50 years ago.

Keep your sucrose intake under control. Not zero, but not a lot. If you keep you carb intake down, this will happen naturally. Avoid a sucrose load on an empty stomach.

Count carbs, not calories

Try to decrease artificial sweeteners. See *Diet and Health* book. They do not work in losing weight and adversely affect the gut biome.

Primarily use stone-ground whole-wheat flour See *Bread in the Modern Diet* book

Here is the pregnancy maintenance diet.

Everyone gets vitamins and omega3 supplements.

With normal weight normal glucose: 150-200 grams carb

With obesity and normal glucose: 125-150 grams

With abnormal fasting or GTT: 75 grams.

Breast Feeding: maintenance diet 150-200 grams

No one gets caloric restriction.

The maintenance diet for normal people has different versions which vary in carb intake.

To prevent T2DM use the normal maintenance one.

If you have a history of insulin resistance, you are on the 125-gram version of the normal diet.

If you have prediabetes, you are on the 50–75-gram version of the normal diet.

If you are on the ketogenic diet, you are at 25 grams or the level that maintains ketones in the urine. You then go on the 125-200 grams normal diet after you have lost enough fat.

Therapeutic fasting 0 calories. This is for special circumstances such as you must lose 15 pounds to get into your wedding dress, or for those who may be considering bariatric surgery. See *Fasting and Autophagy for the Common Man* book.

      All these maintenance diets involve the food engineer who is the primary person in charge of feeding the family. This person decides what food to buy and how to prepare it. A difficult task since for most people there is a certain amount of money set aside for food. The diet must be varied as through history we seem to want variety in the diet. You have many different foods that require many different preparation techniques.

There are different food desires of everyone in the family. You are making food for young children, teenagers, adults, and older people. The meals are usually somewhat scheduled, which means everything has to be ready at about the same time. You are responsible for figuring out how much food to prepare, what food do you have available, food safety, and food storage. There are snacks to be prepared and always special occasions. The food engineer is not the person who decides where you go out to eat every night.

Most people who are obese do not seek advice from their health care provider. I do not blame them. Most start out using their common sense and try to eat less and exercise more. That seems to fail over 95% of the time in the long term. That is why the incidence of obesity is increasing not only in the United States, but also around the world.

Other books by this author

INTRODUCTION FO CELL BIOLOGY AND EPIGENETICS

Paperback Books

Diet and Health

Diabetes, Prediabetes Obesity

Ketogenic Diet for Beginners

Fasting and Autophagy

Maintenance Diet

Bread In the Modern Diet

Epigenetics In Pregnancy

Introduction to Cell Biology and Epigenetics

Diet and Disaster: Food Shortage

Covid and Vaccines for Medical Professionals

Covid and Vaccines for the Common Man

Allulose and Other Sweeteners

Practical Sex for Older Married Couples

Sexuality in Marriage After Fifty

eBook A2 Milk

eBook Brain Disease and Fasting

eBook Tampons and Cancer

eBook Let's Rename PCOS

eBook Weight Loss for Women

eBook-Fat Kids and Fasting

eBook Lipoproteins in Diet and Health

eBook Autophagy and Ages

eBook Carbs for Food Engineers

eBook Fructose and Soy for Food Engineers

eBook Fasting and Disease

INTRODUCTION FO CELL BIOLOGY AND EPIGENETICS

eBook Know Your Orgasm

(for advertising Know Your Organ)

eBook Know Your Masturbation

(for advertising Find Yourself)

eBook Know Your Clitoris

(for advertising Know Yourself)

eBook Artificial Sweeteners and the Gut Biome

eBook 28 Day Fast

eBook Dementia in Women

eBook Fat and Protein for Food Engineers

eBook The Food Engineer

eBook Flour Treatment

eBook Bread Gluten and Sensitivity

eBook Introduction to Stem Cell

(Regenerative Cell) Treatment

eBook Prolonged Fasting

www.ingramcontent.com/pod-product-compliance
Lightning Source LLC
Chambersburg PA
CBHW050005230526
45465CB00003BB/1262